Detox Cleanse Starts with the Colon Cleanse: A Complete Colon

Simple Steps to Colon Cleansing

By: Mary Edwin

I0429841

PUBLISHERS NOTES

Disclaimer

This publication is intended to provide helpful and informative material. It is not intended to diagnose, treat, cure, or prevent any health problem or condition, nor is intended to replace the advice of a physician. No action should be taken solely on the contents of this book. Always consult your physician or qualified health-care professional on any matters regarding your health and before adopting any suggestions in this book or drawing inferences from it.

The author and publisher specifically disclaim all responsibility for any liability, loss or risk, personal or otherwise, which is incurred as a consequence, directly or indirectly, from the use or application of any contents of this book.

Any and all product names referenced within this book are the trademarks of their respective owners. None of these owners have sponsored, authorized, endorsed, or approved this book.

Always read all information provided by the manufacturers' product labels before using their products. The author and publisher are not responsible for claims made by manufacturers.

Paperback Edition

Manufactured in the United States of America

DEDICATION

This book is dedicated to my husband Tom and children Alicia and Rochelle. They have always supported me no matter what the venture. I really could not have a better set of cheerleaders.

TABLE OF CONTENTS

CHAPTER 1- COLON CLEANSE - AN OVERVIEW

Colon cleansing is not just a new fad; it isn't something that Hollywood stars do to lose those extra couple of pounds before their big premier. There are many things that add up to make the colon cleanse benefits worth the time and effort invested.

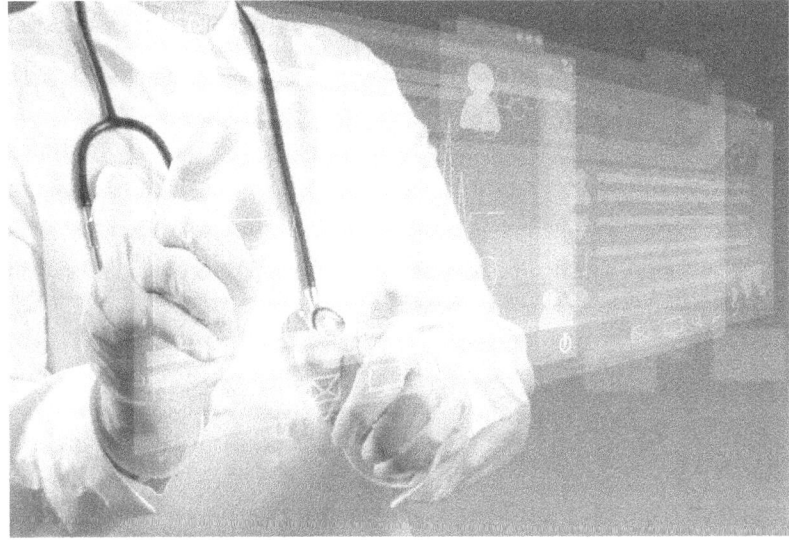

If you are not very regular with your bowel movement, you may be a good candidate for a colon cleanse. You probably don't even know it, but you are putting your body at risk without even understanding the colon cleanse benefits.

Let me start by explaining how this works. Undigested food enters the intestine and basically gets stuck there. So what do you imagine happens with this food once it becomes clogged in your intestines? The fecal matter and food becomes toxic to your system and causes constipation; but can more seriously result in health issues. One of the colon cleanse benefits is that it will release this fecal matter and undigested food that is causing you not only discomfort but also the toxins that can possibly affect your health. Millions of people are suffering from this very thing and often don't realize the colon cleanse benefits.

Fast food, junk food, many refined sugars, diets low in fiber; in general poor eating habits cause your intestine tract to slow down and in effect can cause problems with your digestive system. The sole purpose of the colon is to store waste before it is eventually evacuated from the body, and disruption in this process, or any left behind fecal matter or undigested foods are certainly going to cause problems. When this waste is not evacuated from the system, the toxins are then redistributed into the body, sometimes spreading to the liver and bloodstream. It isn't really necessary to explain the colon cleanse benefits to your liver and bloodstream. These are very important organs that are crucial to your health and wellbeing.

There are many other colon cleanse benefits. Those who are not aware of them often suffer from the poisons that are attacking their system and don't even realize it. Some will suffer mental dysfunctions, joint problems, stress on the heart, skin related issues, etc. Many people have reported weakness in their muscles, tiredness and an overall feeling of sluggishness. The colon cleanse benefits are endless and all the symptoms can be avoided with a simple diet meant to cleanse your system of these toxins.

Obviously the colon cleanse benefits seriously outweigh choosing to not try it especially since it's not an invasive procedure. If you cleanse your colon on a regular basis, (please consult a doctor for the appropriate amount of times for your personal needs) you will be amazed at the difference in your energy level, your weight control and your overall wellbeing.

CHAPTER 2- EVERYONE NEEDS A COLON CLEANSE

When waste builds up in your system and gets into your colon it can become toxic to your body by moving into your blood stream. This often lowers your immune system and makes you more susceptible to illnesses and diseases. A colon cleanse detox is a way to reduce the buildup of such waste as this lowers the toxins in your body. Colon cleansing clears out any accumulated waste, including fecal matter, toxins, dead tissue, parasites, and even yeast infections. Once you have experienced a colon cleanse detox you will be pleasantly surprised by the overall feeling of good health.

When it comes to your body building up toxins several factors determine just how much you have built up in your system and just how likely you are to be a candidate for a colon cleanse detox. First your age plays a big part of it, along with your eating habits, exercise and environment. When it comes to the health of your colon of course a major factor is what you consume. It probably goes without saying, but junk food, fast food and processed foods lead to a greater buildup of unwanted waste and toxins in the system and if this is a big part of your lifestyle, it's likely that a colon cleanse detox is for you.

Are you suffering from bloating, constipation, fatigue, bad breath or body odor? Do you often feel irritable and confused? Then you may in fact be a good candidate for a colon cleanse detox.

Certain over the counter medication like enemas and laxatives can help to cleanse out the toxins in your system, but do not entirely do the job. Enemas and laxatives only clean out the rectum which, as you are probably aware is only a small portion of the intestinal tract.

Detox Cleanse Starts with the Colon Cleanse

When you decide you are in need of a colon cleanse detox you should steer clear of caffeine and alcohol. It's also best to avoid any meat products during a colon cleanse detox. Certain foods are prohibited during the detox phase; however, foods such as fruits and vegetables are not, depending on the detox you have chosen. One key factor in a colon cleanse detox is going to be the consumption of lots of water.

Once you have experienced the wonderful feeling of good health after a colon cleanse detox you will be advising everyone you know to try it too. Your energy will increase, your memory will be better and you may actually end up losing some unneeded weight, leaving you with a stronger more powerful body.

If you're looking for the best colon cleanser, you will undoubtedly be looking for an all-natural colon cleanser. This is because colon cleansing is a process in which the end result is to remove the harmful toxins from your system, this therefore makes it a reasonable assumption that putting unnatural medication into your system will defeat the purpose and ultimately, not achieve the ultimate goal.

The best colon cleanser rids the body of harmful buildup of toxins in your intestinal tract, gives you a great feeling of overall good health and will possibly even help you to shed a few extra pounds.

A natural colon cleanser will most likely consist of some fasting along with a combination of certain ingredients or supplements. You will also most likely see the word Probiotics. The best colon cleanse will definitely have probiotics in it. Probiotics are used to stimulate the liver, gallbladder and intestines. Probiotics increase the growth of the good bacteria in your body, thus helping the process by balancing the good and bad bacteria in your overall system.

Dietary fiber is often overlooked when it comes to bowel disorders and will definitely be seen in the best colon cleansers. Fiber not only helps manage your cholesterol levels but insoluble fiber provides bulk, which in the intestines stimulates the bowels and increases the ability of the intestines to contract, causing the fecal matter to move easily through your system. Psyllium is part of the soluble fiber family and is sometimes called mucilage. Psyllium is often used in the best colon cleansers because it forms a thick gel when it meets water, and in turn allows a more regular flow through the intestines while it helps to remove toxins from the body.

Sometimes a colon cleanse will consist of a diet of strictly raw vegetable, fruits, juice and of course water. But the best colon cleanser will additionally have probiotics, flax seed, bentonite clay and possibly even salt water enemas. Bentonite, if used in a colon cleanser is a form of clay. Bentonite acts like a laxative and removes toxins and parasites from the bowels. Flax seed itself absorbs water and expands in the intestines, further assisting in the removal of toxins from the colon.

These are only a few things to look for when searching for the best colon cleanser. There are many, many options available, but if you are serious about becoming a better, healthier you, it's important that you take it seriously and aim to do it as naturally as possible. Even the best colon cleanser needs the best intentions in order to fully fulfill the expectations. But once you have tried a natural colon cleanser, you too will find yourself telling everyone that you have just found the best colon cleanser!

CHAPTER 3- DIFFERENT METHODS OF COLON CLEANSING

Colon cleanse via the use of commercial products is not the only way to effectively cleanse your colon. In fact, you have two basic types of colon cleansing procedures that you can choose from. Just pick the one that is right for you and you are on your way to regular bowel movements and a healthy colon to boost.

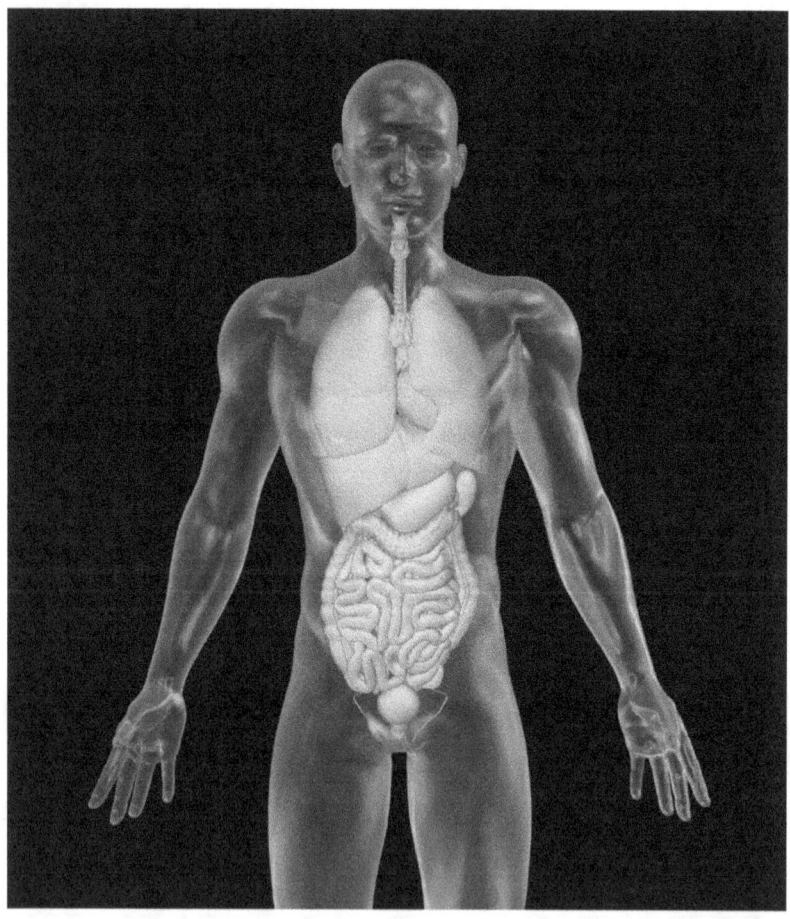

<u>*Colonic Irrigation or Enemas*</u>

Mary Edwin

This is probably one of the oldest procedures when it comes to cleansing the colon. If you have undergone major surgery in the past, then you might have been given and enema to prepare you for anesthesia; you may also have been given one when you were a little kid.

Both Colonic Irrigation and Enemas involve the introduction of water (sometimes a sudsy water solution) in order to irrigate and cleanse your colon. This procedure is also sometimes done to help alleviate flatulence, impacted stools and constipation. Enemas have even been given a bad reputation as something that is only preferred by the elderly.

Nonetheless, enemas and colonics are indeed effective in flushing out the toxins from your colon. But a big downfall of enemas is the fact that they need to be performed by another person and they involve inserting an irrigator into your rectum. Doesn't sound very nice, does it? Well it's not; you would have to spend some time lying on your side with your buttocks hanging out. Not to mention the frequent trips to the bathroom and painful cramping.

But, a good thing about getting enemas and colonics is the fact that they are contained events. You can go for a scheduled procedure, endure a few hours of cramps and bathroom trips, but after that you can go back to your regular routine and you won't have to worry about needing to go to the bathroom at the most inconvenient times. Even if you need to have an enema or a colonic every now and again, you can still find a way to schedule it when you have the time.

Herbal vs. Oxygen Products

There are two basic types of colon cleansing kits; those that use Herbal products as their colon cleansing ingredient and those that use Oxygen. The two products are very different compared to enemas and colonics because they do not involve the introduction of liquid into your colon and (the best part) you can do it on your own and in the comfort of your home. It means that you won't have to visit the clinic, wear a hospital gown, have a nurse irrigate your colon and so on and so forth.

All you have to do is take the scheduled pills and powders and be on your way. The fact that you won't have to make hospital or clinic trips doesn't mean that you are free from the cramping. You will still experience cramping and stomach pains when you use colon cleanse kits – especially herbal ones.

The oxygen powder based colon cleansing method does not have the degree of pain and cramping that the other does, but they still both involve 24/7 trips to the bathroom. Colon cleansing kits are however considered to be much more effective than enemas are; you just have to endure the adverse effects that accompany it.

No matter which procedure you choose, just make sure that it will compliment your lifestyle and give you the results that you want.

CHAPTER 4- THE PHYSICAL AND MENTAL BENEFITS OF HAVING YOUR COLON CLEANSED

Are you considering getting your colon cleansed, but are skeptical about the results that it may produce? One thing you should understand is that colon cleansing is extremely beneficial to your health and you should really consider getting it, especially if you are having problems with irregular bowel movements and are having various gastrointestinal issues.

So, what are the benefits of having colon cleansing? A lot! It ranges from having increased vitality to having better mental clarity. As I said in earlier chapters, colon cleanse or colon cleansing is defined as the process of removing toxins, harmful bacteria (emphasis on 'harmful', because not all the bacteria in our system can cause detrimental effects) and debris. These items can store up in our intestinal canal, especially in the large bowels, due to irregular bowel movement and sometimes improper diet.

Regular bowel movement means that you have one - once a day, or at least six times a week. This means that if your eat a regular diet, but move your bowels an average of only two or three times a week – you are then sure to have a lot of clogged debris in your intestinal canal.

This debris harbors the harmful bacteria and the toxins, which can find their way into your bloodstream and cause innumerable ailments and diseases. That is why you need to have them removed and sometimes the only way to effectively do that is through the process of cleansing your colon.

An Increase In Vitality

Detox Cleanse Starts with the Colon Cleanse

Getting rid of excess debris in your colon immediately makes you feel lighter and less bloated. Plus, the removal of the harmful bacteria and the toxins means that they are no longer reabsorbed into your system and you will feel healthier and have more energy. You would most probably notice this result one or two weeks into the treatment.

Better Digestion

If you constantly suffer from indigestion, flatulence, etc. – a colon cleanse procedure would really help you in this department. Because the process clears your intestinal tract, there is now a much smoother space for your digested food to move through. In order to maintain this result, you now have to advocate for yourself a healthier diet that is high in fiber and fluids.

Increased Mind Clarity

Now, we know you are probably saying: How can cleaning out my colon help me with mind clarity? Well, the answer to that lies in the fact that your intestines have a tendency to absorb into your blood stream the harmful bacteria and the toxins that have logged in your bowels.

These absorbed toxins may then be transported through your blood brain barrier and cause you to have trouble concentrating. Therefore, getting rid of the debris that harbor these toxins would result in you having better focus.

CHAPTER 5- COLONIC USE AFTER COLON CLEANSING

A colon cleanse procedure is intended to remove the toxins that have accumulated in the body. In essence, the buildup of harmful bacteria due to lifestyle choices and dietary options is purged from the system. However, a colon cleansing procedure is not guaranteed to remove all of the toxins located in the body. There are some toxins that still remain that may re-emerge in the bloodstream. This is something that we obviously wish to avoid. It is for this purpose that a colonic is used.

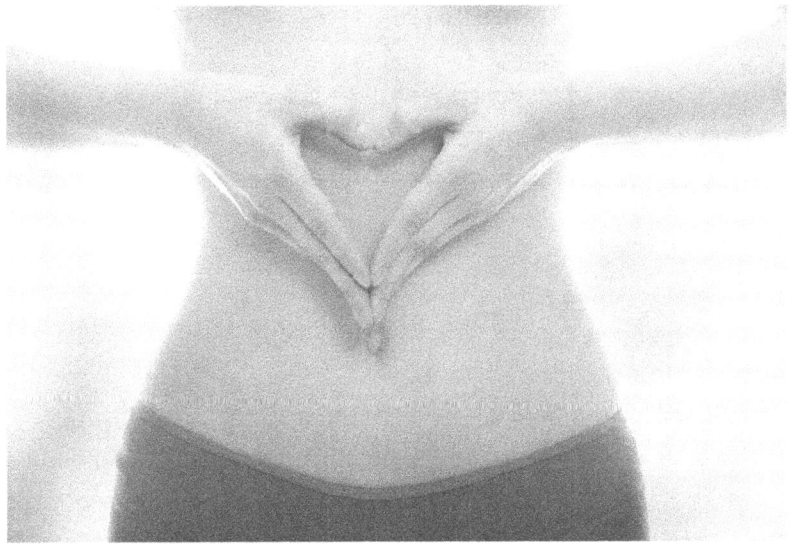

A colonic is more commonly known as colon irrigation or colon hydrotherapy. It involves the insertion of a long tube in the colon. Water will then be circulated around the colon in an attempt to remove the remaining toxins and fecal matter found therein. The colonic process itself is not very painful. Many people liken it to getting a massage for the colon. It doesn't take too much time, either. In fact, a colonic cleansing procedure typically lasts under an hour.

The Benefits Of Colonic Cleansing

There are many benefits of colonic cleansing. The most important is the aforementioned effect of removing excess toxins that remain after a colon cleansing procedure. In addition, other waste and fecal matter that are stuck in the intestinal walls are eliminated from the system.

Another important benefit is the strengthening of the colon. The colonic procedure involves the insertion of water into the system. This will eliminate bulges in the colon to smoothen its shape.

Other benefits of colonic cleansing include improved nutrient absorption, strengthened digestive system, improved energy, lessened mucus accumulation, constipation relief, and clearing of the skin.

Is Colonic Cleansing Safe?

A colonic is a safe procedure. However, there are cases where the equipment used during such a procedure is not cleaned properly. In this case, infections are to be expected. It is therefore imperative to make sure that the equipment used during the procedure is sterilized properly to avoid such an occurrence. Make sure that you look for a credible practitioner so that you would have the assurance of the cleanliness of the equipment.

Before undergoing a colonic procedure, it can be beneficial to take a few precautions. Undergo a fiber-rich diet several days before the colonic procedure. This serves to make the flushing of toxins relatively easy. It is also advisable to drink lots of water and to eat lightly before the colonic procedure.

Mary Edwin

After the colonic procedure, some people experience loose bowel movement. This typically goes away after a few days, so it is absolutely normal. Still, taking a few extra precautions after the procedure can help a great deal. Avoid eating raw vegetables since they are fairly difficult to digest. Instead, get lots of rest and eat light meals.

<u>*A Side Effect Of Colonic Hydrotherapy*</u>

While the real purpose of a colonic treatment is the removal of toxins, it could have the side effect of eliminating the good bacteria in the system. While most of the harmful bacteria are removed during the procedure, the good bacteria cannot be distinguished so it is similarly removed. The use of probiotics is advised to help restore the good bacteria in the system. This helps bring back balance to the system.

Chapter 6- Where To Find A Natural Colon Cleanse Recipe

There are many places to find a decent natural colon cleanse recipe. Many people online have found that certain ingredients assist in making the colon cleanse more effective and have concocted a natural colon cleanse recipe. Some of which are actually pretty good and indeed effective. Below you will find some things to look out for while searching for a good natural colon cleanse recipe.

A good natural colon cleanse recipe that will yield the best results will include things like Psyllium husks or seeds. As mentioned earlier in this book, Psyllium husks offer your colon the bulk it needs to cleanse the waste properly. However, it is important that this be taken will lots of water.

Probiotics are also commonly used in a natural colon cleanse recipe. Probiotics increase the growth of good bacteria that are needed for a healthy system. Any good natural colon cleanse recipe should contain Probiotics, even when purchased from a reputable source.

Potassium is also a factor in a natural colon cleanse recipe. Those that are low in potassium often have weak colon walls, making it harder for the colon to contract and properly move fecal matter through the system. Potassium is also important because in the colon wall tissues it brings in more oxygen, this is very helpful in the elimination of toxins and is very helpful in strengthening the walls along with cleaning out the colon and any excess buildup.

Because of the large amounts of potassium and vitamin A, prunes are an excellent source for a natural laxative. The vitamins in prunes melt down the fecal buildup along the walls of the intestines and help to dissolve blockages while getting the muscles activated correctly in order to remove the waste properly. Other foods that are high in potassium are cabbage, spinach, carrots, broccoli, cauliflower and pineapple. Even if you don't choose to try a natural colon cleanse recipe, it is recommended that you regularly eat a diet high in potassium for the good effects it has on your colon, not to mention the benefit of helping to reduce the chance of constipation. If you can't stomach prunes, it has also been said that pouring hot water over dried prunes and drinking the broth can have the same effects.

Commonly Used Colon Cleansing Herbs

Some common colon cleansing herbs are listed below. You may use some of these colon cleansing herbs in your diet. Most of the herbs listed below are known to have very good effects on the bowels; they help to remove toxins and bacteria from the system and are used to promote proper digestive system function.

As with any major change in your diet it is recommended that you seek the advice of a medical care physician before beginning, especially if you are currently taking other medications, as some colon cleansing herbs can have a negative effect on your body when joined with certain other supplements, or medications.

Aloe Leaf

Although commonly associated with skin care, aloe leaf is also becoming popular for use with improving proper bowel movements.

Bayberry Root

Kills parasites, reduces inflammation, maintains regularity, and boosts the immune system.

Detox Cleanse Starts with the Colon Cleanse

<u>Buckthorn Bark</u>

Softens stools, relieves constipation.

<u>Burdock</u>

Flush excess fluids and toxins.

<u>Cascara Sagrada</u>

Acting as a laxative it is a very well-known colon cleansing herb. Triggering contractions in the colon helps aid in more effective bowel movements.

<u>Cayenne Pepper</u>

Kill parasites. Relieves gas.

<u>Chinese Rhubarb</u>

Along with properties like Cascara Sagrada that trigger contractions in the colon, Chinese Rhubarb also has been known to be helpful for diarrhea and reducing inflammation in the colon which is why it acts as a great colon cleansing herb.

<u>Dandelion Root</u>

Gentle laxative. Antioxidants help remove toxins.

<u>Garlic</u>

Aids in healing, rid the colon of parasites.

<u>Grapefruit Pectin</u>

Removes infections in the digestive system.

Mary Edwin
<u>Magnesium Oxide</u>

Increases hydration to your colon, which helps soften and remove compacted fecal matter.

<u>Peppermint Leaf</u>

Eases pain and aid in removal of infections.

<u>Psyllium</u>

Containing a fiber known as mucilage, Psyllium absorbs water in the digestive tract, making the stools larger and more firm, aiding in more productive bowel movements, making this one of the more popularly used colon cleansing herbs.

<u>Red Clover</u>

Mild laxative and stimulate to the colon.

<u>Slippery Elm</u>

Reduces colon inflation.

These are just a few of the colon cleansing herbs, there are many, many more. If you are not following a specific colon cleansing diet, be sure to do the proper research before taking any herbs and speak to your doctor, as some can be very powerful and also have very negative effects if taken with certain medications.

CHAPTER 7- HERBAL COLON CLEANSE VS. OXYGEN POWDER COLON CLEANSE

As mentioned in Chapter 3, if you are planning to get a colon cleanse procedure it is important for you to understand that there are basically two types of colon cleaning kits that are available in the market today and they are the Herbal and Oxygen type of products. Products from these categories tend to have drastically different results and consumers are divided between the two.

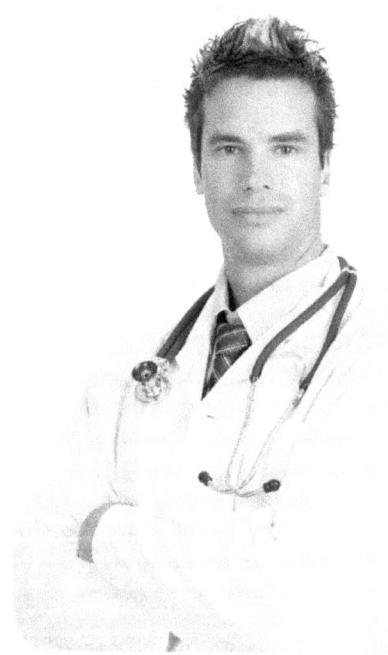

Herbal Colon Cleansing Products

The herbal colon cleansing products work by using a number of well-known herbs that help in the movement of bowel. These products also have added artificial or mild laxatives that help in the elimination of waste.

Mary Edwin

A prominent characteristic of this product are the long mucoid links that are produced by their users. These links are a result of special ingredients that absorb water in the intestines like a sponge. It expands the intestinal walls and gets into the folds and crevices. That way, mucous plaques that may have been attached to walls, literally gets swept away. You need to use these products regularly in order to achieve optimum results.

A downside to these herbal colon cleansing products is that it sends their users to the washroom regularly. The instructions also advocate an increase in fluid intake, so even if you are not having a bowel movement, you would still have to go to the washroom to pee.

Some users have also complained of painful cramping and abdominal aches. But, more or less, herbal products are the most popular in the market because its' users get to see immense results with the mucous stool links that they produce.

Oxygen Colon Cleansers

The oxygen colon cleansers are very different from the herbal products because they do not claim to work from the inside by having expanding fiber like with the herbal products, but instead, they work from the outside with the aid of oxygen.

These products claim that they can cleanse the colon by dissolving mucous plaques through the introduction of oxygen rich blood. This is the same concept as with fat loss through oxygenation.

A good thing about these oxygen colon cleansers is that you would be able to retain your normal bowel movements and you won't have to worry about knowing where the restrooms are. The treatment also claims that the oxygen rich environment created by their products helps stop the growth of harmful bacteria.

Detox Cleanse Starts with the Colon Cleanse

The negative side of oxygen colon cleansers is possibly the fact that they are yet to have dramatic result similar to the herbal ones. They are also more expensive than the herbal ones and some critics say that too much oxygen in the system can cause harm too.

Which Is The Best Colon Cleanser?

Choosing between these two types of products is not easy and you really have to review and research about it closely before deciding on using one in particular. It is also important to avoid making decisions based on testimonies you see on product websites. Try talking to real people, acquaintances and friends who have used the products, and discuss their results with them if possible.

CHAPTER 8- THE PARASITE COLON CLEANSE

It's probably a subject you are uncomfortable discussing and certainly not dinner time talk, but it needs to be said so it can be better understood. Everyone's body is full of parasites, yes, that's right, everybody's body! There it's been said and the voodoo surrounding it can be disarmed. Parasites are especially likely to be found in the intestines and the only way to rid your intestines of these things is a parasite colon cleanse.

Parasites make their way through the system and are a result of contaminated foods and water. Once they enter the colon they begin to attack the system, thus causing infections within the body. Believe it or not, this happens to many people, which is why a parasite colon cleanse is important.

Some typical parasites you can expect to find in the human body are roundworms, tapeworms and flukes. Of course it is very important to detect these worms and get them out of your system which is where a parasite colon cleanse comes in handy and luckily for you, there are many options available when it comes to finding the right parasite colon cleanse for you. Since none of us want these parasites in our system, not to mention the problems they can cause, the only question now is what kind of colon and body cleanse should I do?

Some people choose to rid their bodies of these nasty little invaders by using herbal supplements. Herbal supplements have been known to be effective in removing these pests from the system with very little discomfort, while others prefer to follow a strict diet to flush their system. A strict diet of fresh, raw vegetables, like spinach, tomatoes and carrots, all of which contain anti-oxidants which are very good for the body and help to cleanse the intestines. Yogurt is also a very useful tool for a parasite colon cleanse along with other kinds of colon cleanse and has many useful properties, but most off all helps to balance out the good bacteria.

This may be hard to swallow too, but parasites multiply in very large numbers. One parasite alone can produce thousands of eggs at one time. I know what you're thinking, that you wish you would have heard of this parasite colon cleanse before. I totally understand; it certainly is a disturbing thought. I know it's hard to imagine, and even more disturbing to visualize. This is why it's important to effectively treat with a parasite colon cleanse so they cannot return and of course learn to prevent them from returning in the future.

If you're considering looking into a parasite colon cleanse look for certain herbs to be included, such as sloves, wormwood, and walnut black. These are all very effective in cleaning out the colon and should be included in any good colon and body cleanse.

If you're experiencing any pain you should be proactive immediately, and seek medical attention. Parasites can ultimately cause other health issues and have been known to cause issues such as itchiness, dry, flaky skin and can even dry out your hair. A healthy colon is very important in our overall health and well-being, so take some time to figure out what the right approach is for you and when you're ready you can feel great knowing control is just around the corner and doing a parasite colon cleanse is very much reachable!

Chapter 9- Cleansing The Colon With Laxatives

Colon cleanse is generally a healthy practice. There is no harm in helping the body a little bit in eliminating toxins and trapped waste products in the body.

However, there are some practices that are harmful, according to medical studies. This does not mean that colon cleansing per say is harmful. These studies simply point out that some approaches to colon cleansing are harmful instead of beneficial.

The quandary arises from what is lost during colon cleansing. Since the human digestive system has organs that are interdependent, the system is actually disturbed during colon cleansing.

The "traditional" use of laxatives is to aid people who have problems with bowel movement. Chronic constipation due to dehydration and other problems are remedied by encouraging bowel movement through laxatives.

Many people use laxatives for colon cleansing. The effect of course is increased bowel movement, which might or might not remove significant portions of trapped waste. When a person eats too much meat, enema preparations and laxatives (syrup or tablet forms) are used to help eliminate the indigestible animal material. Bowel irrigation is another colon cleansing approach that uses water to loosen hardened stool from the colon.

Caution Against The Use Of Laxatives

According to Dr. Gabe Mirkin, a practicing internist in Washington, "The human body is so effective in protecting itself from the contents of the colon that enemas and laxatives are necessary only for people who don't eat properly or have a disease that prevents normal elimination."

As you can see, Dr. Mirkin (and many other doctors) disagrees with the use of laxatives for colon cleansing. According to a study published in the Archives of Internal Medicine in 2003, the regular use of laxatives as bowel cleansing agent can cause severe loss of potassium.

Why are doctors concerned with potassium levels? Potassium might be a generally low-profile micronutrient placed next to the popular vitamin family (A, B, C all the way to K). Nevertheless, potassium plays a key role in sustaining human life. Potassium is responsible for the regulation of heartbeat. This is why excessive potassium levels in the bloodstream can cause arrhythmia, angina pectoris or even heart attacks.

The laxative approach to colon cleansing becomes risky because of loss of potassium. In elderly patients, this can affect those with heart conditions.

Why is potassium drained away during the use of laxatives? Sodium phosphate, which is an active ingredient in most commercially available laxatives, is the culprit. The sodium phosphate causes reactions in the body that help expel potassium along with toxins and other wastes. Younger people are generally not affected by potassium loss.

The kidneys of younger people are strong enough to store and retain potassium on their own. However, the same cannot be said for people of advanced age. Older people have generally weaker kidneys. This is a disastrous condition in relation to potassium retention. Since older people are more prone to heart ailments, this is simply unacceptable.

Mary Edwin

Dr. Mirkin suggests that refined carbohydrates be removed from your diet to naturally cleanse your colon. More water is also warranted, to help in elimination.

CHAPTER 10- HOW TO FIGHT CANCER WITH COLON CLEANSING AND ALTERNATIVE DIET

Why do we have to cleanse our colon? For some people, the act is simply a proper way of taking care of the body. Some use natural laxatives like Aloe Vera juice (Aloe barbadensis) and other known natural laxatives.

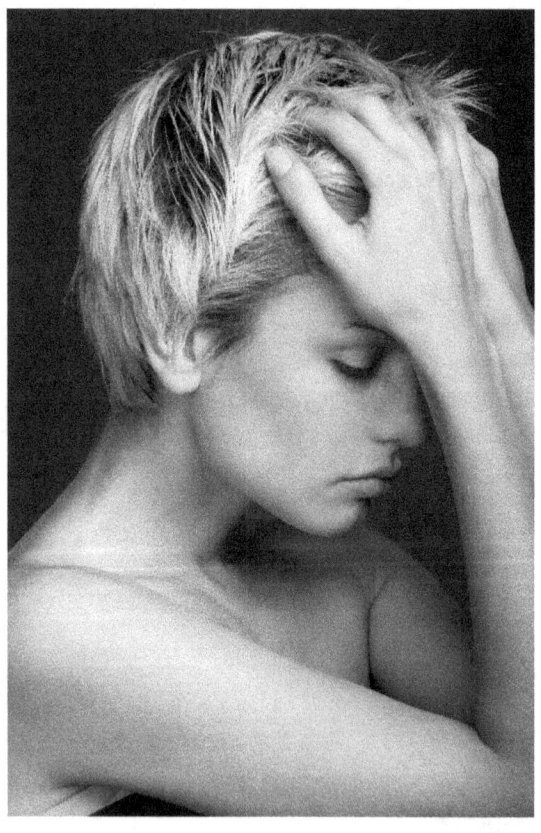

However, did you know that colon cleanse is far more beneficial than what we once thought? Regular and natural colon cleansing helps the body fight cancer even before it forms in the body. A cleansing diet allows the body to repair itself on a daily basis, and allows the digestive system to function more efficiently.

Steps To Cleansing Your Colon Naturally

The first step that you have to make is to stop eating meat. It might sound incredulous, but eating meat has far too many disadvantages. These disadvantages not only affect the cardiovascular system but also place a person in a tenuous position. Bad diet coupled with smoking and heavy alcohol consumption can predispose a person to many forms of cancer, not just colon cancer.

Some may ask, "Can we still add meat as a side dish, or mixed with fiber-rich vegetables?" The answer is still a no. If we are to cleanse the colon completely, protein sources from land-based meat should be eliminated.

If you have been a meat-eater for the past forty years, it would be a struggle to reduce and completely eliminate meat consumption. But it is still worth a try.

People in their fifties to their sixties are predisposed to a host of diseases. Cardiovascular anomalies are just one of a person's problems in advanced age. More insidious and hard-to-detect physiological anomalies abound. These anomalies include bleeding colon polyps and other growths. A lifetime of toxin-rich foods and lack of exercise can take a toll on the colon and the surrounding parts of the digestive tract.

Alternative Protein Sources

Some may think complete elimination is a harsh step. But many people forget that aside from pork, beef and chicken there are still plenty of seafood and fresh fish to choose from. Moving away from land-based animals to water-based animals is a good way of weaning yourself away from meat. It would still be a struggle, since fish and aquatic protein sources are not as filling.

The physiology behind this is the basic fat content of aquatic creatures. Compared to land-based poultry, beef and pork, fish generally has less than 30% fat. Fat coats the stomach, signaling the brain that it has been filled. We feel "full" when this continuous signal is sent by the stomach.

Red meat is a real killer. You should stop consuming red meat as early as you can, as red meat is notorious for low-density lipoprotein (LDL) and a host of other unnecessary and undesirable compounds.

The Connection Between Diet And Cancer

Unsettling as it may sound, our diet has a direct connection to cancer. Persons who have had their bout with cancer know this very well. Cancer patients discover too late in life that their diet had something to do with the cancer they have had the misfortune to have.

Meat makes the body acidic - an environment that allows cancer cells to thrive and metastasize. Meat also provides cancers cells with a form of protein that is directly usable. Eating meat will feed cancer cells. The vital decision that has to be made seems clear.

CHAPTER 11- COLON CLEANSING AND WEIGHT LOSS

As you now know, the colon is part of the large intestine which is responsible for the elimination of waste matter from your body. The health and functioning of your colon plays an important part in your weight loss regime. A healthy and clean colon facilitates weight loss when you are on a diet, while an unhealthy one not only makes you feel weak and ill, it also leads to slower fat and weight loss.

When waste and other fecal matter is stuck to the walls of your colon, you will generally feel fatigued and tired most of the time. Most people are unaware of this, but there is a direct relationship between fatigue and fatigue related ailments like back pains and headaches to a clogged colon. If you are already feeling fatigued, then you will definitely experience problems in following a dieting plan and will not be able to stick to it until the end.

On the other hand, a colon cleanse program will make you feel more energy, vitality and endurance, thus helping you follow your weight loss program to a T.

Cleaning your colon will directly affect your digestion, making it faster and more efficient. When the colon is lined with mucoidal plaque and solid waste, your whole digestive and waste removal system slows down. While this does affect bowel movement at times, unknown to us, the absorption of toxins and wastes into the bloodstream becomes an almost continuous process.

There is a breeding of bacteria and parasites in the colon as well, which causes abdominal pains, flatulence, constipation and other problems in the gastro intestinal system. A colon cleanse on the other hand will clean your colon and get your digestive system back on track, which will make it possible for you to follow your dieting regimen till the end without facing any stomach related problems.

After cleansing your colon, you will experience an increase in both endurance as well as energy while exercising. This will help you in achieving the exercise and workout related goals of your fitness program, thus helping you lose weight faster and better.

What Is The Best Way To A Clean Colon?

While the best way to a clean colon is by consuming a diet that is rich in fiber, this process might not work if you have clogged up your colon through years of taking an unhealthy diet.

Most people consume diets that are low in fiber and complex carbohydrates while being high in fat and sugar content. Apart from this, our dependence on processed food further keeps on clogging all our organs with toxins that are produced as a result of the breakdown of the chemicals and preservatives present in processed foods. It is therefore important that you increase the fiber content of your diet.

In case you have been clogging up your colon through a diet of the above mentioned unhealthy foods for a long time, then it is advised that you undergo a colon cleansing regime in order to clean your colon properly before incorporating diet changes.

Chapter 12- Colon Cleansing Is The Best Cure For Acne

Acne is one of the most common skin problems with a large majority of people all over the world suffering from it. However, there is hardly any permanent cure for acne, especially in allopathic medicine. It is because of this reason that most of us keep trying over the counter lotions and potions in order to treat our acne, but without much success. In order to treat your acne, you first have to understand what causes acne.

The Causes of Acne

We all know that our body has to keep eliminating waste in order to function properly. This is carried out mainly through sweating, urine and bowel movements. However, if the colon and the kidney fail to work properly, then more and more waste is channeled towards the skin, which in turns blocks the pores and causes acne and other skin problems.

Therefore, in order to get rid of your acne, it is important that you go for an internal cleansing instead of taking any kind of medications and creams. Because until and unless the toxic wastes clogging your body leaves it, your skin will keep on erupting.

Clear Your Acne By Cleaning Your Colon

You can cure your acne completely by cleaning your colon, followed by your liver and kidneys. Once your colon is cleansed of waste matter, it will start eliminating waste properly and your skin will stop being clogged by toxins.

One of the best parts about intestinal cleansing is that it can be carried out using natural ingredients that do not have any side effects. This is unlike all the antibiotics and pills that we might take in order to get rid of our diseases. All you need to do in order to cleanse your colon naturally is to take an herbal colon cleanser that can either be made at home or bought readymade online for a week or two according to instructions.

This colon cleanse regime will help your colon in getting rid of all the fecal waste and mucoid plaque that hampers its normal functioning and health. On top of this, there are various ingredients in processed foods that when broken down takes the form of toxins.

Our colon, which is generally overworked due to our trashy diet, is unable to remove all these toxins properly and they find their way to the skin erupting in the form of acne. Once your colon is cleansed, it will be able to remove all the wastes and the toxins that you consume from your body, so the blood that circulates in your body will be pure and free of acne causing toxins.

Many people follow colon cleansing with parasite elimination and liver flushes. All these processes combine to give you a complete internal cleansing, making you healthier and rid of not just acne, but many other diseases. In fact, many people claim that colon cleansing, which has been known to cure all kinds of common acne like rosacea and cystic acne vulgaris is also helpful in healing scars left behind by acne.

CHAPTER 13- HOME COLON CLEANSE

The main goal of an at home colon cleanse is to eliminate the toxins that have laid to rest inside your colon over the years. This can be done safely and effectively in the comfort of your own home. In order to do it effectively you will need to avoid certain foods. Fast food is definitely out the question. Also you should be avoiding refined sugars and junk food totally.

Research has shown that many of us are carrying around as much as 25 pounds of undigested food. 25 pounds. An at home colon cleanse can lead to a healthier, better feeling you. An at home colon cleanse has been known to eliminate some annoying problems such as bad breath, bloating, constipation, diarrhea, fatigue, and some allergies along with many other things that are effecting our daily lifestyles and activities.

Who Is A Good Candidate For An At Home Colon Cleanse?

Do you have trouble with your daily bowel movements? Are you having daily bowel movements? If you're not having a bowel movement every day, if you only eliminate a couple times a week or even every other day, an at home colon cleanse is probably something you should look into.

Typical Things You Can See Without A Colonic Cleanse

Reducing or relieving the symptoms of these conditions are a very big part of colon cleansing and are most definitely colonic benefits that we all would agree are worth it!

- Acne
- Aging
- Allergies

Detox Cleanse Starts with the Colon Cleanse

- Anxiety
- Arthritis
- Asthma
- Bad breath
- Dark circles around eyes
- Extended abdomen
- Fatigue
- Hemorrhoids
- Insomnia
- Memory loss
- Nausea
- Poor circulation
- Sluggish feeling
- Weakness
- Weight gain

<u>Colonic Cleanse Benefits</u>

Along with reducing the above symptoms a colonic cleanse can also aid in:

- Better absorption of nutrients
- Boost in energy
- Clear skin
- Eliminates diarrhea
- Healthier for your other organs, lungs, heart, kidneys, and liver
- Improves digestive system
- Increase immune system
- Lowers the risk of colon cancer
- Lowers the risk of diseases
- No more constipation
- Regular bowel movements
- Relieves acid reflux

Mary Edwin
- Removes toxins from the body
- Rids the body of parasites
- Rids the body of yeast and bacteria
- Weight loss

That is quite a long list of colonic benefits, but it certainly isn't a complete list. Our all over health starts with a good digestive system. Without a well working digestive system, our bodies cannot properly digest and absorb the nutrients correctly, so even though you suffered through eating all your vegetables, your body may not be getting the full advantage of them. After reading the list, I'm sure you'd agree that the colonic benefits are all very important to our overall health and well-being, and that it's certainly worth it.

ABOUT THE AUTHOR

Mary Edwin lives in the country with her family and has always been an advocate for alternate therapies. If there was a minor ailment, she knows which herb could help to solve the problem. She also believes that the body has to be cleansed from time to time to allow it to keep functioning properly. It is the same principle that requires a car to be serviced at a particular time.

As such Mary has written quite a number of books on alternate options to keep the body healthy. Her latest book focuses on the detox cleanse. It is the best way to reset the body naturally.

www.ingramcontent.com/pod-product-compliance
Lightning Source LLC
Chambersburg PA
CBHW070238290526
45789CB00004B/1677